Back Pain Relief:

Home Remedies For Back Pain Prevention
And Exercises To Supercharge Your Health
And Live Pain Free!

Kevin Hughes Copyright © 2015

Table of Contents

Introduction

First and foremost I want to thank you for downloading the book, "Back Pain Relief: Home Remedies For Back Pain Prevention And Exercises To Supercharge Your Health And Live Pain Free!"

In general, we often take our backs for granted until it's already too late and we become injured. When exercising we often make the mistake of only focusing on our arms and legs in order to enhance our appearance. It's time to change all that!

This guide will go over prevention techniques, home remedies and exercises one can use in order to live pain free and get back to doing the things you love to do on a daily basis.

In this day and age the majority of us are now sitting in the car for hours a day commuting back and forth to work, then sitting at our desks for 8 hours a day of work, followed by sitting in front of a computer or TV for hours on end once we get home at night.

Over time this can wreak havoc on the health of our back and lead to some painful and chronic back injuries. It is my hope that you can take the knowledge found in this book and apply it to your lives in order to avoid these common pitfalls.

Thanks again for downloading this book, I hope it helps!

Chapter 1: Common Causes of Back Pain

For most of us back pain can seem like something that is unavoidable. However, you're actually in better control of it then you'd imagine.

There's countless ways to injure your back during the course of a normal day but here are four of the more common causes that stand out.

1. ***Thinking you're invincible..*** What I mean by this is many people will jump into any activity without thinking about the possible consequences. From finishing a few labor intensive chores around the house to playing a game of basketball or tennis. Over time these types of activities can begin to cause a lot of wear and tear on your back and lead to injury. It's not only important to stretch before doing strenuous activity but to incorporate some back exercises into your normal workout schedule in order to strengthen the muscles in your back. Building up your obliques and side abdominal muscles are crucial for the long term stability of your back. If you don't like weight training then try yoga or pool exercises. Another idea is to get an inflatable exercise ball you can sit on instead of always using a chair. As a bonus there's a ton of exercises you can incorporate an exercise ball into.

2. ***Improper Lifting Techniques..*** Bending improperly and then lifting is a major cause of back injuries. Instead follow these few steps to improve your technique.

   • Bend at the knees and be sure to keep a straightened back. Do not bend from your waist.

   • When lifting keep whatever objects your lifting in close proximity. The farther away the object your holding, is from you, the more stress you place on your back.

   • Don't hold the item your lifting above your armpits or

below the knees.

- Try and avoid moving something that is over 25% of your actual weight.

- When lifting don't turn, twist, or pivot. Instead, keep you feet pointed at what your lifting, and stay facing it while you lift. Always be sure if you're going to change your direction, to do it with your feet, instead of the waist.

3. *Carelessness During Day To Day Activities*.. It's often the simplest of things that can cause the most damage. Something as innocuous as washing dishes, or emptying garbage can wreak havoc on your back and twist your spine if you're body isn't properly prepared.. Personally, I once threw out my back taking a dish out of the lower section of my dishwasher. It's not always lifting or moving the heavy items that will do us in. That is why exercising your back and abdominal muscles are such an important thing. You need to keep the core muscles of your body in shape to help ensure long term health. One good simple exercise to incorporate is pulling your navel in towards the spine, as you try and imagine you're wearing something tight that is pulling in the sides of the abdominal muscles.. You can do this a few minutes a day and it'll help make a world of difference over time.

4. *Driving & Sitting in General*.. Long periods stuck in the car, or on a train, to and from work can do an incredible amount of damage to your back over time. The discs inside your back are spongy and help to cushion vertebrae in the spine. Unfortunately, these disc also have a bad blood supply. When sitting still for long periods of time you're actually depriving the discs inside your back of the nutrition they require to function and remain healthy.. The more sitting you do, the more damage you inflict on these discs over time, and the more it stresses the entire back. Be sure to always take

breaks every hour in order to stretch and get blood flow going.

Chapter 2 – Basic Standing Tips

In this chapter we will be talking to you about how you should stand. Most of us don't realize how we stand affects our posture, feet and leg health as well as how pressure on our shoulders will affect our lower back. Read these tips and apply them to your everyday life.

TIP #1 - DON'T LOCK YOUR KNEES

Locking your knees when you stand is a terrible thing to do. When locking your knees, you're putting pressure on the joints in your knees, as well as blocking off an artery that supplies blood flow through the body. If you do this for a long time there is a slight possibility that you could pass out from it.

TIP #2 - PUT YOUR FOOT ON A LOW STOOL

To alleviate back pain it's a good ideas to place your foot on a low stool when standing. There is something known as swayback that occurs when you stand. This is when you have a protruding abdomen or slumped shoulders. To avoid this it is recommend that you help your posture by placing one foot on a low stool to adjust for your weight dispersal.

TIPS #3 - AVOID STANDING IN THE SAME POSITION FOR AN EXTENDED PERIOD OF TIME.

It is a common practice in our work environments to stand in the same place for an extended period of time. When we do this we don't' exercise our muscles, and as a result, we can start to become stiff. Jobs like security guards, doormen and others that require we stay in one place for a long time are among the most affected. If you find yourself in this position, it is highly recommended to take breaks, or stay active to keep your muscles loose and the blood flowing.

TIP #4 - AVOID LEANING BACKWARDS

When standing you will want to avoid leaning backwards. When you lean backwards you will be putting extra strain on your lower back. When you lean backwards your center of gravity is shifted causing your spine to compress and pinch nerves.

TIP #5 - DON'T LEAN FORWARD

Leaning forward is just as bad as leaning backwards. You are moving your center of gravity forward causing stress and strain on your lower back. Doing this for prolonged periods of time can cause damage and irritation to the joints, muscles, and ligaments in the lower back. If you do need to lean forward, do it carefully, making sure to bend your knees in the process so that you limit any damage that may occur

Chapter 3 – Basic Walking Tips

Walking is a crucial part of our daily lives. Walking, is in general, our main form of transportation. When you get up in the morning you walk from the bed to the bathroom, around your home getting ready, to the car to get to work, and then out and about through the course of your day. With all of this walking it is no wonder that we tend to over exert our bodies. In this chapter, I will be giving you tips on how to improve your walking and how to lessen the impact on your lower back.

TIP #1 - AVOID HIGH HEELS AND OTHER HARD SHOES

High heels and hard soled shoes are more of a fashion statement than a requirement to walk. When wearing these shoes you are putting stress and pressure on your legs and feet. As a result it affects your posture, which in turn, adds stress to your muscles in the back. If you are required to wear these shoes try to do it on as limited a basis as possible.

TIPS #2 - WATCH YOUR STEP

It is very important to judge the height of curbs, stairs and other obstacles in your path. Putting too much effort in trying to traverse a step, curb or other obstacle can cause your leg to come up too high and come down hard causing shock and injury to your body. If you under estimate the distance or height you can cause yourself to trip and fall. Be careful not to come down hard on your legs when you walk because you may over judge the height, or cause your foot to get caught, causing you to fall and hurt yourself.

TIP #3 - OPEN DOORS WIDE ENOUGH

Make sure that you open doors wide enough to fit through. You don't want to twist and turn your back to fit through a narrow opening. Doors are designed to fit people through with room to spare. If you are carrying a package or moving something through a doorway, be extra careful, in order to avoid strain on your back.

TIP #4 - MILITARY STANCE

One great tip is to walk as if you were in the military. I know what you are saying, but simply put, it's the best way to walk for the long term health of your back. You'll want to pivot feet first and then the body. This is the best way to move from a standing position.

By doing this you are not putting any stress on your body when you move. The weight of your body all moves in uniformity. At the same time you'll be evenly distributing your weight to all pressure points at the same time.

In this chapter we have briefly discussed some of the points that you should be looking at when you walk. The most important thing that you should remember is to take it easy and don't rush. You don't want to cause an injury by doing something that could have easily been avoided. Make sure to do stretches every morning in order to get your muscles and back limber and ready for the day.

Chapter 4 – Basic Sitting Tips

In this chapter we will discuss how sitting can affect your lower back. We don't realize that when we slump in our chairs we are putting pressure on our lower backs as well as our shoulders. The softness and hardness of the chairs we sit in also affect our backs. Read the tips that I present to you in this chapter and apply them to your life.

TIP #1 - SITTING IN THE CHAIR

When at home or at work you will want to choose the right chair that best suits your needs. The chair shouldn't be too hard or too soft. You'll want to choose a chair that has a firm back to it. You'll want to avoid low overstuffed chairs if at all possible. Chairs should be used for working not lounging.

TIPS #2 - SIT WITH YOUR SPINE FIRMLY SUPPORTED

When you choose your chair you will want to make sure that you choose one that firmly supports your spine. You don't want to have a back that is too loose that it causes you to lean backwards as well as one that is too ridged that doesn't allow for any movement at all. Before deciding on a permanent chair you'll want to try some out on a trial basis to see how they affect you.

TIP #3 - AVOID SITTING IN THE SAME POSITION FOR LONG PERIODS OF TIME

Just like standing in the same place for a prolonged period of time, sitting in the same place for an extended period of time is also not good for you. When you sit in the same position for a long period of time your muscles will begin to get stiff and the fluids in your body will begin to settle. When you have to sit for a long period of time you may want to consider scheduling breaks. These breaks will allow you to get up and moving in order to get the blood flowing through your body.

TIP #4 - AVOID CHAIRS THAT HAVE ROLLERS

You will want to avoid chairs that swivel or have rollers on them. Depending on your environment this can be a safety issue. Chairs with rollers can easily get caught on a rug or rip in the floor as well as topple over if leaned back on or pushed in the wrong way.

In this chapter we reviewed several different things to consider when sitting. Since this is an activity that most of us take part in on a daily basis, in front of the television and computer, it is very important that you choose the right chair for the each situation. Also, don't jump onto the next big trend in chairs or get the one that fits your grandmother. You'll want to take your time and test out a few different options when it comes to choosing the one that is just right for you.

Chapter 5 – Basic Driver and Passenger Car Tips

In this chapter we will be discussing how to protect yourself from back pain while sitting in a car, either as a driver, or the passenger. Most of us spend at least two to three hours a day in our cars, driving back and forth to work, running errands or just getting out for a nice leisurely drive. We don't really think of the damage we are doing to our backs and body in general. In this chapter, I will give you some tips that you should follow and apply to your daily life.

TIP #1 - GET IN AND OUT OF YOUR CAR WITH YOUR BACK STRAIGHT

When you enter your car or exit your car you will want to do it with a straight back. You don't want to squeeze yourself in or try to get in or out at odd angles. The right way to get into your car is to place your right hand on the hood of the car and you're left on the door. Move your body into the car at a 15 degree angle as to mimic the angle of the seat. Once you clear your head you'll want to gradually move your feet into the car, plant them firmly on the ground and close the door.

Once this is completed make sure that you fasten your seat belt and adjust your mirrors. You'll want to make sure that your entire body is aligned within the operations specs of the car for optimal vision and comfort. Also, you want to sure you can comfortably reach the gas and brake pedals while seeing clearly in every possible direction.

TIP #2 - ADJUST THE CAR SEAT

The drivers chair should be firmly positioned for optimal use. The back of the chair should be at an angle that is both comfortable for the driver, as well as allow them to see all around themselves through both the mirrors and the windows.

The seat should also be positioned close enough to the steering wheel in order for the driver to be able to reach both the gas and break. When someone enters the driver's seat they must encompass themselves in a world that is both comfortable and optimized for safety. If the car is ever used by a different driver they must adjust all of the preexisting mirrors and seats for their optimal usage.

TIP #3 - FASTEN YOUR SEATBELTS

Fastening your seat belt is not only the law it is a good way to ensure that your body stays in a fixed but movable position. When you wear your seat belt the belt allows you to move around in the chair but also allows you to keep a standard posture. If you don't wear your seat belt you'll begin to lean to one side or lean forward in your seat. This is not a desirable position.

TIP #4 - GET OUT AND STRETCH

When you're on long trips you'll want to get out of the car every few hours to stretch and loosen up your muscles. Just like sitting at work or standing, like we discussed previously, the same applies when you're riding in a car. You'll don't want to be sitting in the same position for hours on end. Not only will your muscles begin to ache but your concentration will begin to waver.

TIP #5 - TAKE A SMALL PILLOW

When you travel long distances, or are going to be in the car for an extended period of time, you may want to consider taking a pillow and placing it between your lower back and the car seat. This will give the driver extra support and comfort while on those long drives. It will also help you when you pull over at a rest area for a quick cat nap.

TIPS #6 - MAKE SURE YOUR DRIVER IS AWAKE

As a passenger in the car it will be your job to keep the driver awake. To do this you'll need to be comfortable as well. When sitting in the passenger seat of the car make sure that your knees are bent not stretched out. If you're short in stature you may need to bring along a small box or something that can be placed on the floor to rest your feet upon.

TIP #7 - PLAN YOUR ROUTE BEFRE YOU GO

Make sure that you plan your trip before you go. You will want to make sure to travel roads that are smooth and will not jar the car causing unwanted pressure or strain on your back. You will also want to watch traffic conditions to ensure that you're not sitting in traffic jams for hours on end.

Chapter 6 – Back Pain Symptoms and Signs... When You Should See A Doctor.

There are wide ranges of different ways to injure the back. Here I'll go over some of the symptoms of back pain to watch out for. These symptoms can often range from mild to excruciating in intensity.

Symptoms May Include:

1. Pain that begins to radiate from the lower back down to your buttocks and into your thigh, calf and even toes.

2. Sharp pain in a specific area of the body such as the upper back, neck or lower back. Can often occur after improperly lifting a heavy item, or over exerting yourself physically. Upper back pain is sometimes also a sign of an impending heart attack or other major condition.

3. Chronic aching in the lower or middle back due to standing or sitting over an long period of time.

4. Unable to stand up straight without experiencing muscles spasms or pain in the lower area of the back.

5. Constant stiffness or aches along the spine, from the tail bone up to the base of your neck.

Call a Doctor About Your Back Pain If:

1. Your pain begins to increase if you bend forward from the waist or while coughing. It may be a sign that you've herniated a disc.

2. You experience tingling, weakness, or numbness in the legs, arms or groin. This could mean you've possibly damaged your spinal cord.. Immediately seek medical supervision.

3. You experience pain that goes down from the back, into the back of your leg. In this case you could be suffering sciatica.

4. You notice a fever, or frequent and burning urination to go along with your back pain. This could be a sign that you're suffering from an infection.
5. You begin losing control of your bladder or bowels while experiencing back pain. Immediately seek medical supervision.
6. Some other areas of concern include dramatic weight loss, a history of previous trauma, a history of previous cancer, pain lasting for more than a month, pain that does not subside after you've rested and night time pain.

Chapter 7 – Yoga For Back Pain Exercises.

One of the easiest and most effective ways to eliminate chronic back pain is to practice a few back strengthening yoga exercises every day. Here I'll go over a few great yoga exercises to help you beat that back pain that's been keeping you from fully enjoying your life.

These moves will help strengthen your core and back. It is recommended to do functional training such as shown down below on an average of 2 to 3 times each week for between 20 and 30 minutes at a time.

The great thing about these exercises is that they can be performed just about anywhere. Just be careful to keep close attention on how your form is during each exercise. Remember, it only works if you do it properly. Form is key! Also, try to repeat each of the exercises between 2 and 4 times in order to reap the back strengthening benefits.

WARMUP

Decompression Breathing: Breathing in some extra oxygen can really make a world of difference, especially when you're lengthening your body. This move will help show you how to better breathe deeply, and also how to keep your spine strong and long all the time.

First stand with toes touching and keep your heels apart slightly. Shift your weight onto your heel, then unlock the knees while gently pulling both of your heels toward one another. Be sure to stand up tall, keep arms stretched high overheard, and your fingertips pressed together. When you inhale also lift your rib cage out away from your hips. When exhaling begin to tighten you core in order to support your lengthened spine. Keep repeating these breathing techniques and process until you're feeling supported and tall.

YOGA EXERCISES FOR BACK PAIN

I'm not going to bore you with lengthy descriptions on each of these exercises. I find when performing yoga it's best to learn by watching visual instruction. Form is a key factor in yoga and I find it can sometimes get lost in written translation. These exercises are all easy to search for and find on sites like YouTube. You don't need to incorporate all of them into you're routine but you should do a little research on each and determine which one's would best suit your particular set of circumstances.

A.) Neck stretch

B.) Roll on back

C.) Knee hug

D.) Reclining twist

E.) Bound reclining twist

F.) Cat cow

G.) Cat pose press

H.) Tail wag

I.) Hip rolls

J.) Triangle pose

K.) Lunge

L.) Active lunge

M.) Lunge hip opener

N.) Sitting forward bend

O.) Serpent partial lift

P.) Elbow serpent

Q.) Sitting twist

R.) Corpse pose

Chapter 8 – Ten Back Pain Stretches & Exercises

Taking the time to learn a few effective, safe stretches and exercises is a great way to relieve chronic back pain. Always be sure to consult your physician before undertaking any new exercise regiment. In this chapter, I'll touch on ten great stretches and exercise you can easily incorporate into your daily routine. Feel free to mix and match whichever one's make the most sense for you.

Stretch #1: Extension

Begin by lying face down with both feet fully extended behind you. Next lift up your head. Follow this up by arching your back and support the upper portion of your body with only your arms. Keep your elbows locked straight and keep your hands at your side in order to better accentuate your stretch.

Stretch #2: Rotation Stretch

This is intended to stretch all the muscles that help rotate the back. To accomplish this sit comfortably while turning only your shoulders in one direction while holding the position. Using an exercise ball is a great tool to enable you to do this stretch effectively and comfortably.

Stretch #3: The Sideways Bend

This stretch is also done in the seated position. To begin, clasp both hands together then extend them overhead. Keep the arms extended and bend your entire upper body over to one side while holding the stretch. Next repeat this stretch in the other direction. Again, using an exercise ball is a great tool to enable you to do this stretch effectively and comfortably.

Stretch #4: The Hamstring Stretch

These stretches are crucial to any proper back stretching regiment. Correct posture depends both on how flexible your back is but also on the muscles linking your other extremities with your back.

There are many ways to perform this particular type of stretch. A simple way that I prefer to use is sitting, with a leg extended, while the other leg is kept folded inward. Next, reach down slowly to touch your toes on the extended leg. Switch legs and repeat the process.

Exercise #1: The Ab Crunch

Strengthening your abdominal muscles is an often overlooked yet incredibly important group of muscles to focus on when working to alleviate back pain. Begin by placing both feet on something like an exercise ball (I prefer the exercise ball because it really helps to hone the workout without ever straining my back). Next, place hands behind your head and perform a sit-up. That's all there is too it.

Exercise #2: The Exercise Ball Crunch

Using the exercise ball helps to accentuate the effectiveness of your crunch on the abdominal muscles. Start by laying with your back firmly on the ball and your feet on the floor. Next, using only your abs lift both your shoulders and head. When both of these are lifted, hold the position instead of going back down.

Exercise #3: Planks

These can be done either with the exercise ball or without. Lie down face first, then push your body up, balancing with only the toes and forearms (if you're using the ball then on your shins instead of tocs). The key part of doing a plank properly is holding the torso as rigid as possible without your butt stuck up in the air.

Exercise #4: The Press

Doing a bench press can help exercise both the shoulders and upper back. First lie down on something that supports your back (bench or exercise ball both work). Don't concentrate on the weight you're pressing, instead the important thing here is your control and form. Press upwards while at the same time contracting the ab muscles and keeping your back supported.

Exercise #5: Dumbbell Row

For this exercise I suggest using an exercise ball. Ir's not necessary but I prefer it for the support it provides while doing the exercise. Also, as with the press exercise don't concentrate on the weight you're pressing, instead the important thing here is your control of your movement and form. First lay front down on your ball. Hold a pair of weights straight down without your arms locked. Next, bend your elbows and pull up both weights until your elbows have become level with your torso. Be sure to keep the shoulders relaxed. Lower the weights and repeat for between 1 to 3 sets consisting of between 10 to 16 reps.

Exercise 6: Bicycle

This exercise should always be gradually started. Lie on your back and fold both arms behind the head. Next, bring down one of your elbows to your opposite knee. Relax, then bring the other elbow to the opposite knee. As you begin to get used to the process, speed up until you begin the resemble the motion of a bicycle being peddled.

Chapter 9 – Home Remedies For Back Pain

Ice:

Simply applying ice wrapped in a protective covering (to prevent ice burn) or a cold pack is still among the best pain relieving treatments available. When applying ice do not do so for more than twenty minutes and only apply a maximum of ten times during the course of an entire day.

Icing is most effective on minor injuries such a muscle pulls or back strains.. Ice calms down inflamed and swollen tissue.

Heat:

Apply heat for between 15 and 20 minutes.. Moist heat is superior to dry heat. When using heating pads do not set on high.. Always use the low or medium settings. Also do not fall asleep while using a heating pad in order to avoid burning yourself accidentally.

Heat is most effective for chronic pain or stress related back pain. Heat is good for soothing our central nervous system, and allowing relief from fear and stress, which play a factor in many chronic back pain issues.

Massage:

This is a major way to help treat back pain. Many studies show the significance having a routine massage can make, depending on the type of back pain your experiencing. Each type of pain requires different techniques so it's important to do a little research on what kind of massage would work best for your set of particular issues.

Acupuncture:

Studies on this technique are mixed but personally I know people who swear by it. The majority of research I've seen suggests that acupuncture provides some beneficial relief and only a small chance of any negative side effects. Personally, having needles stuck in my back doesn't sound appealing but what works for me is bound to be slightly different then what might work for you. I would always seek out a well trained professional for the best chance of success with the method.

Diet:

You are the things you eat. There are a good number of foods that actually help reduce inflammation; and on the flip side, also foods that increase it. When suffering from back pain it's important to choose foods wisely.

Keeping a diet revolving around plant based foods, like chia seeds and flax, is your best chance to keep inflammation at bay, especially, when you eat these combined with fish like mackerel, salmon, herring, tuna, black cod and trout. Other foods to consider are vegetables like spinach, kale, broccoli, beets, and carrots. Protein like chicken, beans, turkey and cocoa are important. Spices like cinnamon, basil, ginger, garlic, rosemary, oregano, turmeric and cumin are great for seasoning.. Be sure to drink water, or true teas and herbal teas like white, oblong and green tea.

Make sure you're getting enough calcium in your diet. It's easy to overlook this but bone mass decreases as we age and calcium helps contribute to maintaining and forming bone mass. A lack of calcium can lead to other back and bone conditions like osteoporosis.

Some of the foods to avoid include fast foods, saturated fats and processed foods. These foods all help to increase inflammation. This means try to also avoid pasta, white bread, rice, snacks or drinks high in sugar, alcohol and caffeine.

Aroma Therapy:

There are many essential oils that are great for relieving pain and soothing aching backs. Some have properties that are anti-inflammatory and help to reduce inflammation while others are analgesic, and help to reduce pain. There are also oils that have antispasmodic and anti-rheumatic properties..

Here is a list of some essential oils I recommend checking out... The one's that may be right for you will of course be determined by your particular set of back issues.

Important:

Some oils are not suitable for women who are pregnant and some oils should not be used in concert with certain medications. You should always consult a doctor before beginning treatment.

1.   Thyme – An antispasmodic. Great for muscle and joint pain. Also good for a backache.

2.   Chamomile – An anti-inflammatory. Great for relieving spasms and muscle pain. Also good for lower back pain and headaches.

3.   Lavender – An anti-inflammatory. One of the most popular essential oils. Great for relaxation and pain relief. It also has sedative and anti-microbial properties. Does well on spasms, muscle tension, allergies headaches and joint pain.

4.   Sweet Marjoram – A sedative. Good for relieving stiffness, spasms, muscle pain, osteoarthritis and rheumatism.

5.   Eucalyptus – An anti-inflammatory and analgesic. Good for nerve pain and muscle pain. Should only be used in small increments.

6.   Rosemary – An antispasmodic and analgesic. Good for headaches, back pain and muscles pain.

7.   Peppermint – Good for nerve pain, joint and muscle pain.

8.   Sandalwood – A sedative. Good for sedating the nervous system which helps to alleviate nerve pain and muscle spasms.

9. Clary Sage – An anti-inflammatory and antispasmodic. Helps at easing muscle tension and spasms. Use only in small increments.

10. Juniper – An antispasmodic. Good for relieving muscles and joint aches, spasms and nerve pain.

11. Yarrow – An analgesic. Is a strong restorative and pain reliever that is great for joint aches, muscle soreness and pain.

12. Ginger – Good for improving mobility and easing back pain. Good for rheumatic and arthritic pain. Also good for sprains and muscle pain.

13. Frankincense - An anti-inflammatory. Helps at alleviating stress and also serves as a gentle sedative.

14. Vetiver – Good for muscular pain and general back aches.

15. Wintergreen – Good for nerve pain, headaches and arthritis.

16. Helichrysum – Expensive but valued as an antispasmodic, anti-inflammatory and analgesic. Great for quick pain relief and supporting our nervous system.

While it's possible to use these oils individually, it can also be good, to blend as many as 3 oils together. Before applying dilute first with something like jojoba oil, sweet almond oil or olive oil.
You can apply the mixtures in a variety of settings. From soaking in a bath tub, getting a relaxing massage, to using with a hot / cold compress. I would try different oils and different applications to find the ones that best suit your needs.

Herbal:

Research into herbal remedies is in it's infant stages. There are quite a few herbs that are believed to decrease inflammation and ease pain. It's important to be careful and proceed with caution.
Here a few common remedies for pain relief.

1. Capsaicin – Made from hot Chile peppers, this is a topical that can be used to help relieve pain. Its slow acting and can sometime for the effects to be noticed.

2. Feverfew – Used in the treatment arthritis and body aches. Avoid if pregnant.

3. Turmeric – Used in relieving inflammation and pain. Try to limit your dosage and do not use if suffering from gallbladder disease.

4. Devil's Claw – Good for lower back issues and arthritis. Do not take if pregnant or if you suffer from ulcers or gallstones.

5. Valerian Root – For muscle cramps and spasms.

6. St. John's Wort- Good for sciatica and arthritis.

7. Kava Kava – Good for neuropathic pain and tension headaches.

Medications:

Many people will often resort to trying pain relievers before seeing a physician, or pursuing other avenues of back pain prevention. It's important to remember everything you've tried including what worked and what didn't. It's also crucial to keep track of what you're taking as certain medications don't interact well with other medications.

Some back pain relief medications include:

1. Acetaminophen – Commonly found in Tylenol. Safe in normal doses. Helps with pain relief.

2. NSAIDs (Non Steroidal Anti-Inflammatory Drugs) – Commonly found in ibuprofen (ex. Advil, Motrin), and also found in naproxen (ex. Alleve). Great for the treatment of pain affecting muscles and bones… Better than acetaminophen for back pain relief. Not suggested for long term use as they can lead to dangerous long term side effects.

3. Narcotic Painkillers – Prescribed by a doctor, and include oxycodone, codeine, morphine and hydrocodone. These come with many side effects, like possible constipation, confusion, sedation, nausea, urinary retention and allergic reactions. These can also quickly become habit forming. Good only as prescribed for short term use.

4. Muscle Relaxers – Commonly found in carisoprodol (ex. Vanadom, Soma) and cyclobenzaprine (ex. Flexeril). These focus in on the muscles instead of our central nervous system. Only use under close doctor's supervision as they can become habit forming.

5. Adjuvant Medication - Not normally prescribed for pain relief, they're usually prescribed along with other types of drugs to be used in combination for back pain relief. Often used in pain related to our nerves. These can include beta blockers, anticonvulsants and antidepressants.

6. Anesthetics – Work by blocking affected nerves that surround our spinal cord. Can come in over the counter topical creams, or in local anesthetics, like lidocaine and novocaine that need to be administered.

7. Steroids – Used to treat back pain brought on by inflammation. Should not be used for longer than a couple of weeks as they can cause long term complications.

Water Therapy:

Exercising in a pool is a great way to help with back pain. Water buoyancy supports a bunch of your weight making it simpler to move around and improve flexibility. Water will also add resistance to your movement, in turn strengthening muscles. Pool exercises will also help to improve balance, agility and overall fitness. Pool exercise is also great for sufferers of back pain, arthritis, joint replacements and a host of other health issues. Exercising in a pool also helps to reduce the risk of falling and injuring yourself.

Before beginning any new exercise routine always consult your doctor to make sure these pool exercises make sense for you. Here are a few tips to help you get started.

1. Use water shoes. They will help provide more traction on the floor of the pool.

2. Water can be either chest or waist high.

3. Use a flotation vest or belt for deep water.

4. Slow movements offer less resistance, in comparison to faster movement.

5. Don't keep pushing through if feeling any pain.

6. Webbed gloves made for water or inflated balls can help to increase resistance.

7. Keep hydrated. Even though you're in a pool your body still needs water.

6 Pool Exercises:

1. **Side and Forward Lunge**s – Do this near a pool wall in order to support yourself. For forward lunges take a huge step forward and for side lunges take a huge step to your side. Don't let your forward knee go past your toes. Begin with three sets of ten lunge steps.

2. **Water Walking / Water Jogging** - In waist or chest high water, walk 15-20 steps forward, followed by the same backward. Over time build up speed until jogging. Then alternate between walking for half a minute and jogging half a minute. Continue at least five minutes.

3. **One Leg Balance** – Keep standing on just one leg while raising your other knee up to hip level. Hold for around thirty seconds and then switch legs. Try two sets of five on both legs.

4. **Sidestepping** - Face towards pool wall. Then take a sideways steps using your body as well as your toes facing the wall. Take around twenty steps in one set direction and then switch to the other direction. Go twice in both directions.

5. **Hip kickers** - Stand at the pool wall with one side of your body there for support. Then move your one leg forward keeping your knee straight, as if you were kicking. Then begin again at your starting position. Next move that same leg to your side, and again return to your starting position. Finally, move the same leg, but this time behind you. Repeat for three sets of ten and then change the kick leg.

6. **Arm Raises** – Use webbed gloves or a set of arm paddles to add resistance, and keep arms held at your side. Then bend

both elbows to ninety degrees. Next raise and then lower both your elbows and your arms down towards the surface of the water, while still keeping the elbows at the bent ninety degree angle. Do three sets of ten.

There are many other fields of study and therapies for helping to relieve back pain.. Beyond the obvious of losing weight and getting better sleep here is one more alternative to consider.

Talk Therapy:

Still a new field but some studies suggest that Cognitive Behavioral Therapy (CBT) can have long term positive effects on those suffering chronic lower back pain. If you want an alternative option to normal medicine this may be an avenue to research further.

Conclusion

Well I hope that you enjoyed going through this book of back pain tips. Hopefully you'll take away something from it to apply to everyday life. Through my years of experience I have found that following these simple tips and applying them to your lifestyle will greatly decrease your level of pain and allow you to live a happier life.

Education and exercise is key to keeping our bodies safe and healthy. If we just take a little extra time to treat them right, they will treat us right in the long term.

Thank you again for reading this quick e-book. I wish you all the best in health and happiness.

www.ingramcontent.com/pod-product-compliance
Lightning Source LLC
Chambersburg PA
CBHW060347290526
45791CB00004B/1571